Apple Cider Vinegar & Baking Soda 101 for Beginners

BJ Richards

Disclaimer

Legal Notice: - BJ Richards and the accompanying materials have used their best efforts in preparing the material. This book has been composed with the best intention of providing correct and reliable information. The information provided is offered solely for informational purposes and is universal as so. This information is presented without contract or any type of guarantee assurance.

BJ Richards makes no representation or warranties with respect to the accuracy, applicability, fitness or completeness of the contents of this book. The information contained in this book is strictly for educational purposes. Therefore, if you wish to apply ideas contained in this book, you are taking full responsibility for your actions.

BJ Richards disclaims any warranties (express or implied), merchantability, or fitness for any particular purpose. BJ Richards shall in no event be held liable to any party for any direct, indirect, punitive, special, incidental or other consequential damages arising directly or indirectly from any use of this material, which is provided "as is", and without warranties.

Any and all trademarks used in this book are owned by the owners themselves, are not affiliated with this book and for clarifying purposes only.

As always, the advice of a competent medical, legal, tax, accounting or other professional should be sought. BJ Richards does not warrant the performance, effectiveness or applicability of any sites listed or linked to in this book. All links are for information purposes only and are not warranted for content, accuracy or any other implied or explicit purpose.

This book is not intended as a substitute for the medical advice of physicians or veterinarians. The reader should regularly consult a physician or veterinarian in matters relating to his/her health or the health of their pet and particularly with respect to any symptoms that may require diagnosis or medical attention.

ISBN: 978-1-7324365-4-1

Dedication

Thank you, Carl, for all your support.

And to my little fur children for keeping me sane.

Contents

Introduction

Why are you here? And why this book?

Probably, you've heard all the buzz about apple cider vinegar and want to find out if it's true. You've been online going through the thousands of articles and are overwhelmed with trying to figure out what's what and who has the most accurate information.

You want to know if ACV can help you with your issues. You may be dealing with diabetes or gas and bloating. Or maybe, you want to lose weight and you're tired of all the expense and inconvenience of trying thing after thing and getting nowhere. You want something natural that doesn't cost a fortune and can get you some help sooner, rather than later.

If that's the case, then you're in the right place.

I'm going to give you the facts, as best I know them, with several ways to start using ACV today. So, no more waiting and no more nonsense.

There are hundreds of articles and books out there and it can be daunting trying to go through it all. Well, now you don't have to. I've done it for you. So, keep reading and welcome to the word of Apple Cider Vinegar (ACV).

Chapter One

Apple Cider Vinegar as A Super Food

In this chapter we'll cover what raw apple cider vinegar (ACV) is and some of the main reasons it can be such a boon to your health.

The list of super foods is growing. A super food contains a high number of essential nutrients that when consumed regularly, can have a positive effect on your health. Hardly a week goes by without another super food being championed by the media.

Why do we need super foods? In a nutshell, the typical diet is low in essential nutrients. Manmade processed foods are convenient and easily available but tend to be low in essential vitamins and minerals. Without vitamins and minerals, your body won't function properly, and your health is likely to suffer as a result.

Super foods such as pure cocoa, blueberries, green tea, spinach and maca are promoted as having amazing health qualities, but the newest (and probably the oldest!) super food is raw apple cider vinegar.

So, just what is apple cider vinegar?

Natural apple cider vinegar (ACV) is made by crushing fresh, apples and allowing them to mature in wooden barrels. The sugars in the apples then ferment and turn into wine. As the apples ferment further, they become vinegar. The word vinegar comes from the medieval French term "vin egre" and it literally means sour wine.

The primary ingredient in any vinegar is acetic acid. It is an effective natural bacteria fighting agent that contains many vital minerals and trace elements such as potassium, calcium, magnesium, phosphorous, chlorine, sodium, sulfur, copper, iron, silicon, and fluorine, which are vital for a healthy body. All vinegars also have other vitamins and nutrients. The concentration depends on what the vinegar is made of.

ACV has been around for centuries and was used in cooking and medicine. Manufactured from fermented whole apples, the best apple cider vinegar is raw. That is to say, it has not been pasteurized, distilled or filtered, as these processes can reduce the healthful properties of the vinegar.

Also, raw apple cider vinegar that has been correctly processed contains what is called the "mother". The "mother" is that muddy looking substance that settles to the bottom of the bottle. This is where the enzymes are that give you the great health benefits. So, you only want to buy apple cider vinegar that says it contains the "mother" on the label. This is also why you always want to shake the bottle before you pour any for use. You want to be sure you're getting this good mother substance evenly distributed throughout the rest of the liquid before you use or consume it.

Raw apple cider vinegar is best purchased from health food stores rather than grocery stores. This is because the vinegar sold for cooking is lower quality than the vinegar made for consumption as a health supplement. When it comes to apple cider vinegar, it pays to read the label and get the best product you can find. There are numerous excellent products on the market. Bragg's Raw Apple Cider Vinegar is probably one of the most well-known, but there are a number of other reputable ones as well.

An Age-Old Remedy

For centuries, apple cider vinegar has been used as a medicinal remedy for a number of illnesses.

Some of the old-time uses for ACV are killing warts, fighting infection, as an antiseptic and even to increase fertility!

Since there were no studies done back-in-the-day, it's hard to say if this super food really helped any of those conditions. But, there is no doubt it can be useful for improving general health and helping with weight loss in particular, as well as other situations we will cover later on.

ACV is nutrient dense. Nutrients are vital for health. Without nutrients such as vitamins and minerals, your cells, organs and bodily systems will not function properly, and ill health is likely to follow.

Modern diets are often low in essential nutrients and many people eat too much processed food. Processed food, as the term suggests, has been through a refining process to change the taste, texture and/or shelf life of the food. That often leads to few or no healthful nutrients surviving those strong chemical processes.

Many people's diets are very high in calories but low in essential nutrients, so even an overweight and clearly overfed person can be suffering from malnutrition.

Consuming raw apple cider vinegar is an easy and convenient way to get a daily dose of essential nutrients.

So what nutrients does this powerful food contain? It's quite a long list and as long as you're consuming raw apple cider vinegar, not processed, you'll be giving your body a good dose of the following

- Vitamins A, C, E, B1, B2, B6, K
- Beta carotene (a form of vitamin A)
- Potassium
- Calcium
- Magnesium
- Phosphorous
- Copper
- Iron

There aren't many foods, raw or otherwise, that can boast such a side variety of nutrients!

According to a study published at HealthLive.com (https://www.healthline.com/nutrition/apple-

cider-vinegar-weight-loss#section4)
apple cider vinegar has been shown to:

- Increase metabolism (the rate at which you burn calories)

- Decrease appetite

- Reduce fat storage

- Lower blood glucose levels

- Improve fat burning

You've just learned how to obtain wonderful results from an inexpensive and readily available source! Now, let's find out how to use this amazing resource in the next chapter.

Chapter Two

How to Use Apple Cider Vinegar

In this chapter we'll cover how to use apple cider vinegar, so you can start getting its benefits right away.

Like anything else, there are things you should know before ingesting something new.

Make sure never to consume ACV without first diluting it in water using a 10 to 1 ratio, i.e., 10 parts water to 1-part ACV. There are a couple of reasons for this. The first being, ACV is very acidic and can burn the delicate tissues in your mouth, gums and throat. The second is, due its high acidity, taking ACV straight can damage the enamel on the teeth. Always rinse your mouth and brush your teeth after taking it, even diluted.

Also, don't get stuck in the mindset that a little is good, so more is better. Too much ACV taken incorrectly can result in decreased potassium level and bone mineral density.

(https://www.karger.com/Article/Abstract/4518
0).

Always consult your health care professional
before starting a new regime, especially if you're
taking medications. ACV may interfere with
certain blood thinners, laxatives, heart disease,
diuretics or diabetic medications. Pregnant
women, nursing women and people with chronic
health conditions should consult their doctors
before starting an ACV regimen.

If you suffer from any of the following, you may
need to avoid ACV completely: low potassium,
Barrett's esophagus, hiatal hernia, ulcers. Again,
consult your health care professional first so you
know if this is something for you.

If health is your aim, you should consume one
diluted teaspoon of apple cider vinegar first thing
in the morning, (but not on an empty stomach)
and last thing at night. This will ensure you get a
good nutritional start to your day and provide
essential nutrients for the repair process that
happens while you sleep. You can eventually
work this amount up to one tablespoon per day if
you choose.

If you are interested in weight loss or appetite
suppression, consume one diluted teaspoon of

ACV 15 minutes before all main meals. For most of us, this means one teaspoon three times a day. We'll cover more on this, as well as the maximum daily dosage, later.

If you are feeling hungry between meals, you could also try a diluted teaspoon of ACV to ward off an unruly appetite. As well as preventing hunger, this means you get an extra shot of healthy vitamins and minerals.

Apple cider vinegar is a 100% natural product and is safe for a vast majority of the population to use. Not only is it safe, it can help with numerous medical conditions including:

- Arthritis
- High blood pressure
- Circulatory problems
- Depression
- Indigestion
- Digestive upsets
- Headaches
- Nasal congestion

- Rashes

- Ulcers

That being said, you should never attempt to self-medicate with ACV and should always discuss your medical requirements with your family physician. It's unlikely your doctor will tell you not to take this food, but it's always best to check and make sure.

You should be aware that ACV has a few mile side effects, including stomach upset. Furthermore, ACV may worsen heartburn in some individuals. It is also known to thin the blood and should be avoided by anyone taking blood thinning medications such as anti-coagulants.

Providing you doctor gives the all-clear, you might find that your condition and symptoms improve rapidly soon after you start taking apple cider vinegar.

It's clear that this super food is healthy and useful for fat loss, but only if you actually move from reading to doing. There are so many other ways ACV can benefit you and your family. It's relatively cheap, easy to obtain and could be one of the best things you do for your health.

Now that you know how to use ACV, let's get specific about those health benefits. We'll talk about that next.

Chapter Three

Health Benefits of Apple Cider Vinegar

In this chapter, we'll go into detail about how ACV helps you maintain your health.

Apple cider vinegar has been called a cure for almost everything. Health enthusiasts have used it for everything from acne and allergies to sore throats and warts. Vinegar in its many forms has been used for centuries for all sorts of folk remedies. Recently, with the flood of people turning to home and natural based remedies, apple cider vinegar has come to light as an especially useful health tonic.

People are often skeptical about something as common as ACV's ability to be an effective treatment for so many issues. Folk remedy experts have long used it as a natural cure-all. Recently though, research conducted on the proposed benefits of ACV have proven many claims correct.

Perhaps this is why Oprah (http://bragg.com/blog/index.php/all-natural-organic-whole-live-foods/tag/oprah-show/), CNN (https://www.cnn.com/2017/04/18/health/apple-cider-vinegar-uses/index.html), and CBS (http://newyork.cbslocal.com/video/3562948-health-trend-apple-cider-vinegar/), just to mention a few, rave about apple cider vinegar and its benefits.

Here are some of the major benefits many have experienced with apple cider vinegar:

- Weight loss aid

- Acid reflux reduction or elimination

- Acne relief

- Wart elimination

- Heartburn relief

- Kill yeast infection

- Arthritis pain reduction

- Improve skin appearance

- Cholesterol control

- Improve hair strength, density and luster

- Blood pressure control
- Sinus infection relief
- Kill candida
- Gout relief
- Body detox
- Dandruff elimination
- GERD relief
- Relieve constipation
- Diabetes control

We've just covered a brief overview of ACV and its many uses. With its many benefits, it's no wonder why a lot of people are talking about apple cider vinegar and what it can do your health.

Next let's take a closer look at how apple cider vinegar can assist in weight loss and appetite suppression.

Chapter Four

Apple Cider Vinegar and Weight Loss

We've all heard the buzz about ACV and losing weight. This chapter will help explain why.

Do apple cider vinegar weigh loss plans work? That's the question many people want to know. For years, people have looked for ways to lose weight. They have tried all kinds of things, some that worked and some that didn't. apple cider vinegar has shown real promise when it comes to losing weight and keeping it off.

Using an apple cider vinegar weight loss plan isn't new. People have been using ACV for this purpose for decades. One reason it continues to resurface in popularity is because the weight may come off more slowly than many of the fad diets, but it also tends to stay off, which means control of yo-yo dieting, cravings, and the never-ending fad diet trials.

There have been several studies on the subject of weight loss and ACV, some of which were quoted earlier. Part of what ACV does to help with weight loss centers on diabetes and insulin resistance.

Diabetes is when your body doesn't produce enough insulin to deal with the sugar levels in your blood. Insulin resistance is a step lower than diabetes. Your body is still producing the right amounts of insulin, but that insulin is less effective at lowering your blood sugar levels than it should be.

ACV can help lower blood sugar levels. This helps your body process the remaining glucose with the insulin produced. When your body can't process the sugars you take in, they get stored in fat cells. That causes you to gain weight.

Taking in too many calories, sugars, or anything else will cause you to gain weight. Part of the problem it that not everyone can recognize when they feel full. So, they just keep eating and eating, until they feel physically full. But there have been studies that suggest people who take a little ACV with their meals feel fuller faster.

There are a number of versions of the apple cider vinegar diet.

Most of them suggest you start with 5-10ml (1 to 2 teaspoons) per day and gradually increase to

30 ml (2 tablespoons) per day. Going beyond 30 ml (2 tablespoons) per day is generally not recommended.

One version calls for you to have 1-2 teaspoons of ACV diluted in water before every meal. It's supposed to help you feel fuller faster. It also helps to regulate the time it takes for the glucose produced from your foods to reach your bloodstream. Having the release of blood sugar regulated means your body won't have to produce as much insulin. The less insulin your body produces, the less it triggers your body to start producing fat cells and storing fat. That will help you lose weight.

Below is a more detailed description of how ACV breaks down fat, revs up the metabolism and helps you lose weight.

Helps to Reduce Cholesterol Level

Bile is a viscous yellowish liquid produced by the liver that helps to break down dietary fats and dispose of leftover cholesterol and other toxins from the liver. Poor bile production hampers liver activity, which may result in accumulation of fats and cholesterol, adding to obesity. Consuming one diluted teaspoon of ACV early in the morning kick-starts bile production, promoting fat breakdown and cholesterol decomposition.

Lowers Blood Sugar Level

A spike in the blood sugar level increases the cravings for snacks and unhealthy processed foods, which is a big turnoff if you're trying to shed a few pounds. According to published studies (https://www.healthline.com/nutrition/6-proven-health-benefits-of-apple-cider-vinegar#section3), apple cider vinegar helps to lower blood sugar levels. The results were that those who drank ACV diluted in water before a meal had lower blood sugar levels than those who did not.

Aids in Blocking Carbohydrates (Starch)

Gone are the days when it was believed that carbohydrates are bad for your health. The new age of dieticians recommends consumption of carbohydrates regularly to ensure a balanced diet.

The starch contained in carbohydrates tends to convert into glucose quickly and stimulate the release of insulin in the body. The insulin triggers the storage of glucose in the form of fat. Hence, eating starchy food pushes your body into the fat storage mode.

The acetic acid content in the vinegar interferes with the body's ability to digest starch. It helps to reduce the storage of glucose in the form of fat. Over time, this starch blockage activity will have an effect on body weight reduction.

Promotes A Healthy Digestive System

Your gut contains trillions of probiotics (healthy bacteria) that help to break down complex food particles. This combats the growth of disease causing microbes and regulates the immune system. ACV acts as a catalyst for these probiotics. The probiotics feed on the pectins contained in apple cider vinegar for growth and development. Hence, ACV helps to maintain optimum gut flora for smooth digestion and body metabolism.

Suppresses the Appetite

Apple cider vinegar contains pectins, a type of soluble fiber that provides a feeling of fullness to suppress the appetite for all the good reasons.

Acts as a Mild Laxative and Diuretic in Nature

ACV acts as a mild laxative to accelerate the elimination process and ensure regular bowel movements. It also has a diuretic effect, helping to release excess stored water from the body.

Promote Body Detox

Body detoxification refers to the thorough cleansing of the body to get rid of accumulated body waste, such as undigested food, cholesterol, saturated fats and disease-causing microbes. Due to an unhealthy diet and/or poor lifestyle habits, body metabolism slows down and body toxins start to pile up.

The combined effect of the sluggish body metabolism and accumulated body toxins can result in obesity. ACV is a detoxifying elixir that is natural and safe. It promotes digestion, speeds up body metabolism, relieves constipation and excretes excess water from your body to cleanse it from the inside.

The benefits of ACV for weight loss are obvious., But, ACV should not be considered a miracle cure. Combining ACV with a healthy, low-calorie diet, a positive attitude and regular physical exercise will yield the highest results.

We have just learned how ACV helps get rid of unwanted weight and keep it off.

Now let's look at how ACV helps relieve of the biggest problems many face today... heartburn and indigestion.

Chapter Five

Heartburn, GERD and Acid Reflux

This chapter is about excess gas that comes from poor digestion. We'll explain the terms above so it's easier to understand.

Heartburn, GERD and acid reflux aren't different terms for the same thing. But they are closely related.

Acid reflux is when stomach acid flows backward into the esophagus. The specific term for it is gastroesophageal reflux. If this happens to you, you'll probably get a taste of regurgitated food in the back of your mouth or experience a slight burning sensation in your chest.

As acid reflux gets worse, it progresses into GERD (gastroesophageal reflux disease). One of the common symptoms of GERD is frequent heartburn.

Heartburn is a symptom of acid reflux and GERD.

So, the question is, does using ACV help with these issues? Or is this just another one of those old wives' tales. Keep reading and let's find out.

As you know, ACV contains minerals as well as trace elements. Due to all of its beneficial ingredients, ACV is a natural fighter of bacteria, which often makes it an acid reflux treatment of choice.

Why? The reason is digestive problems like acid reflux are not caused by too much acid but too little (https://chriskresser.com/what-everybody-ought-to-know-but-doesnt-about-heartburn-gerd/).

Apple cider vinegar mimics the acid level of the stomach, which aids in the proper digestion of food and can help aid the stomach in digesting its contents.

This is why ACV works more effectively than antacids. Antacids can help heartburn, but they are designed to diminish acid within the system. This means antacids will not treat the actual cause of acid reflux. Instead, they can make reflux more frequent.

Recipe for Relief

When taking ACV, you want to shake it well before you ingest it to disperse the sediment and stringy materials at the bottom throughout the liquid. This is where the greatest concentration of vitamins and minerals lie.

To start, try taking one teaspoon of ACV diluted in a glass of water before each meal. ACV is an acquired taste. You should grow more accustomed to the flavor after the first few ACV acid reflux doses.

Nevertheless, should you find it too repellant, there are a few other ways you can take ACV, such as:

- Mix a tablespoon of ACV with a fat free salad dressing or light mayonnaise and eat it with your meal.

- Sprinkle a tablespoon of ACV on salad or vegetables.

- Mix a teaspoon in an 8 oz glass of water and add a bit of honey to sweeten the drink and neutralize any acidic after taste.

- Make a tea out of ACV by adding a teaspoon of the it to hot water and slowly sipping it.

Although it is best to ingest ACV prior to each meal, you can take a teaspoon diluted in water when your stomach is upset or heartburn acts up.

As we learned earlier, it's best to start slowly and build up from a teaspoon to a maximum of two tablespoons per day. And always dilute it in water if drinking instead of mixing into food.

After taking ACV for a few days, many acid reflux sufferers find their symptoms improve and continue to improve with treatment in the months that follow. Always remember you should speak to your doctor before starting any new health regimen, including ACV for acid reflux. Keep in mind that natural regimens should not replace any medication or treatment advice prescribed by your doctor without prior consultation.

We've just explained the different types of unwanted gaseous upsets most people experience from poor digestion and how you can help yourself with ACV. Next, we'll cover the widely discussed top of diabetes and how ACV can help there.

Chapter Six

ACV and Diabetes

Now, let's find out how apple cider vinegar deals with diabetes. That's what this chapter is all about.

Many diabetics who are interested in a diabetes remedy has been asking about ACV. Though there are many types of alternative treatments, ACV is one many people turn to.

Each week, thousands of diabetics try simple treatments and lifestyle changes to try to reverse and sometimes cure their diabetes. If you're interested in an alternative diabetes therapy, ACV has a lot to offer.

Its potential impact in the fight against diabetes has increasingly become the subject of many studies. As the evolution of modern lifestyles has led to a perceptible increase in the incidence of this disease, man has started to look for different ways to deal with it. The sumptuous carbohydrate-rich diet of modern man, consisting of bread, pasta, pizza and grains, is said to be one of the major causes of the prevalence of diabetes.

This search for cures and preventatives has led to rediscovering the health benefits of such natural remedies like apple cider vinegar.

In today's world, diabetes has become a leading cause of mortality worldwide. Diabetes is an ailment where wayward elements of the body's defense mechanisms attack the pancreas. As the pancreas produces the sugar-regulating hormone insulin, any attack renders in incapable of defending against sugars that normally accumulate in the system. If blood sugar levels increase at a rapid pace and remain unregulated, there can be damage to blood vessels and vital organs like the brain. Once these vital parts are damaged, secondary diseases and ailments may develop, and these are typically considered 'diabetes complications'.

There are two types of diabetes: Type 1 and Type 2. Type 1 diabetes, also called juvenile diabetes, is where the pancreas is unable to produce adequate amounts of insulin. It is normally treated via insulin management. Type 2 diabetes, often called adult onset diabetes, is where the body is no longer responsive to insulin produced by the pancreas. It is treated in a variety of ways.

Preliminary studies conducted in the United States have found that taking apple cider vinegar may help lower the rise in blood glucose levels after food intake. It is said that the high acetic acid content in apple cider vinegar may help slow the digestion of starch, thereby reducing the glycemic or glucose index of starchy foods.

A small study of Arizona State University researchers and published in the *Diabetes Care Journal* (http://care.diabetesjournals.org/content/27/1/281.full), showed that people who took apple cider vinegar with their food before bedtime showed remarkably reduced glucose levels in the morning.

Advocates of apple cider vinegar who use ACV, encourage people to look for Raw, unfiltered, unpasteurized versions, as opposed to processed vinegars available in big stores and supermarkets.

Analysts also say vinegar dietary supplements in capsule or tablet form may not be as effective for managing blood glucose increases after meals. The tablet form doesn't contain acetic acid, the primary gent for controlling blood glucose levels. It is best to use raw apple cider vinegar for this purpose, properly diluted in water.

How to Take

When using apple cider vinegar to control diabetes, start the regimen slowly and gradually work your way up. The typical way to consume ACV for blood glucose control is to put two teaspoons of ACV into a glass of room temperature water and drink before meals. When taken in this manner, the ACV will help control the sugar spike when food is taken in.

Diabetes patients need to inform their doctor if they plan to use apple cider vinegar to help control their condition. There might be some medications that have been prescribed that could have counter effects with the vinegar.

We've covered the many benefits of ACV and how that can help diabetes. Next, we'll talk about your skin and the benefits apple cider vinegar can help you with there.

Chapter Seven

Acne and Apple Cider Vinegar

In this chapter, we'll discuss acne and ACV can help. We'll cover other skin applications you can benefit from, as well.

You may have heard this saying, "An apple a day keeps the doctor away". Well, today, I'm going to tell you something different: "Apple cider vinegar each day keeps the acne away".

Out skin is naturally acidic. Our skin needs that acid mantle to protect itself from bacteria and germs. But we often disrupt that acidity by using harsh soaps or cleansers. ACV works because it restores the needed acidity to our skin, allowing the skin to protect itself from pollution and germs once again. It also removes the oil, dirt and dead skin cells that contribute to clogged pores and acne.

Apple cider vinegar is able to break down excess fat, mucous and phlegm, thus improving the health and function of your liver, bladder and kidneys. The liver and kidneys are the main organs in your body that serve to detoxify and cleanse.

As you know, acne is usually caused by accumulated toxins in your body pushing through the pores in the skin. By taking ACV, you help your body rid itself of these unwanted toxins. ACV is also antibacterial. It is this antibacterial property that directly assists your skin in cleansing itself and healing the acne outbreaks.

What to Do

Here is a home remedy for acne you can try. Mix 2 teaspoons of ACV in a glass of water and drink it once in the morning. If you find it hard to drink, try adding some honey to sweeten it. This regime will handle the internal application.

For the external use of ACV on your skin, try this toner.

First be sure to shake the raw apple cider vinegar well so you're getting the sediment of the mother solution at the bottom distributed throughout the bottle.

Then, mix about 1 tablespoon of the ACV in 2 or 3 tablespoons of water. The more sensitive your skin is, the more water you'll want to use. You'll have to experiment to find the right dilution for you. I recommend starting with a more diluted solution to make sure you're not over-drying your skin.

Next, apply the toner solution you've just created and wait for it to dry completely. After that, apply whatever lotions etc., you usually use. Do this twice a day or whenever you wash your face.

Another great facial treat is a bentonite clay mask using ACV in the liquid used to mix the clay in.

If this is your first tie using bentonite clay and ACV on your face, start with a once-a-week treatment with this mask. If it works for you, try increasing the use of the mask to twice a week, etc. Some even do it every day, but you don't want to start there. Once a week in the beginning is best.

There are two types of bentonite clay: sodium bentonite clay and calcium bentonite clay. Most people use the sodium bentonite clay for detoxing and the calcium bentonite clay for remineralization. I recommend the calcium bentonite clay for this. There are many different brands out there. You'll want to read reviews and see which brand is best for you.

Here are some of the great benefits you can expect from this mask:

- Helps prevent acne breakouts and clean up existing ones

- Draws out debris and toxins from the pores.

- Helps to heal and rejuvenate your skin.

- Helps to reduce the intensity of scars.

- Shrinks pores and unclogs them.

- Blackheads seem to disappear.

- Is a great natural exfoliant.

- Gently evens out skin tone.

- Leaves your face feeling soft with a natural glow.

For this recipe you'll need:

- 1 teaspoon of bentonite clay

- 1 teaspoon of apple cider vinegar

- 1 shallow glass/dish/cup, etc.

Put the bentonite clay and apple cider vinegar in a shallow dish and mix with clean fingers into a paste. If you use a spoon, don't use a metal one. The metal elements from the spoon will leach into the clay and you'll reduce the effectiveness of the mask.

If you find the mask is too strong or too thick, add a little water to the paste. You want a paste that will spread easily, so you may need to play around with adding more clay or water to get it where you want it.

Now apply the mask to your face. Many also apply to the neck or upper chest. You can use your fingers or a cotton ball or clean cosmetic sponge. Apply a thick layer.

It will take about 15 minutes for the mask to dry if your application is thick. You'll feel your skin tighten as the mask dries.

Leave the mask on about 20-30 minutes in the beginning. You can extend the length of time you choose, but only after you've used the mask several times and know your skin type and how it reacts to the mask.

After the allotted time has passed, rinse off the mask with plain water. You'll probably need to use your fingers to scrub it off in some places, as it has a tendency to stick.

Your skin will likely look a little pink right after you rinse off your mask. This usually only lasts a few minutes and happens to everyone. That's because as the clay pulls out the toxins, it increases the blood flow to the face.

If your skin is sensitive, try using a thinner application layer of the paste and leave it on a shorter period of time. After you see how your skin reacts, you can use a thicker paste layer and leave it on longer. Do this gradually to make sure you're finding the right combination of mask layer and time for your level of skin sensitivity.

I've just shown you how to make an effective facial toner and clay mask using apple cider vinegar. But what about your hair? We'll talk about that next.

Chapter Eight

Dandruff, Hair Loss and Weaves

In this chapter we're going to talk about your hair. We'll be covering the main issues most people are interested in: Hair loss, thicker more lustrous hair, dandruff and weaves.

Almost everyone is looking for ways to make their hair thicker without it costing a fortune, especially if dealing with thinning hair or hair loss. ACV has been a great help with these issues for thousands of people.

Because ACV is so full of nutrients, it has the ability to balance the pH of your scalp. Plus, it helps to remove the dead skin cells that clog up the follicles and stunt the hair's ability to grow.

We've talked about the high acidity in ACV due to the malic acid. When you add the powerful enzymatic nature in the mother part of ACV, you end up with something that will kill a germ called "bottle bacillus". This germ is often responsible for many hair elated maladies, including thinning hair and even baldness in some cases.

Bottle bacillus can clog up the hair's ability to secret the natural oils our hair needs. That means the hair starts to starve and then fall out or break since it's not getting the nutrition it needs. The result is hair that starts to thin and break easily. This, unfortunately, can lead to baldness.

So how do you use ACV to help prevent all that and start your hair back on its recovery to being full and shiny?

<u>Try this hair rinse:</u>

Make a 1:1 mixture of raw ACV and water. It's great to make a little extra so you have it ready ahead of time. Use a 16 oz plastic bottle and put 1 cup of raw ACV and 1 cup of water in it.

Now shampoo your hair as your normally would. Then gently rub in the ACV rinse you made. You want to leave it on for 5 minutes then rinse thoroughly with water. Some also like to do a deep conditioner after. Give yourself a nice scalp massage while you're at it. The 5 minutes will go by quickly that way and your scalp will love it.

For Dandruff

You'll be doing almost the same procedure if you're dealing with dandruff.

Mix ¼ cup ACV and ¼ cup water and spray your hair thoroughly after shampooing. You can use the hair rinse you've already made in you want to.

Massage it into the scalp and let it sit for 15 minutes, then rinse.

Do this twice a week and you'll be rid of the dandruff before you know it, all without having to resort to expensive chemical-laden treatments.

ACV for Weaves and Extensions

Apple cider vinegar is amazing at bringing the hair used in weaves and extensions back to life. When you purchase high quality virgin hair the cuticles are intact and fully sealed. No chemicals have been used so the hair is nearly perfect. However, as soon as you start using shampoo, coloring, hot curlers, etc., the cuticles will begin to strip down until you have unmanageable hair that's just sitting on top of your head. That's what happens to your extensions, too. Using ACV brings the pH balance back to its normal level, thus rejuvenating your hair, including the hair you use in weaves and extensions.

So, how much apple cider vinegar do you need? This ratio is a little different than what was discussed earlier. Here you'd want to use 3 parts water to 1-part ACV. Put the clean hair in a large bowl containing this mixture and leave it for 45 minutes to an hour. If your hair is on your head, shampoo first, then put on the mixture and put a cap on to cover your head for the same amount of time.

When the time is up, rinse out the ACV and use a deep conditioner. Conditioning the hair plays a big role in the outcome, so don't cut corners. A little time will save you the cost of buying new hair so often.

When you're done, you will find your hair is sleek, slick and beautiful, just like when you first got it.

Now that you know how to beautify your hair, let's talk about a number of other ways ACV can help in your daily life.

Chapter Nine

Additional Uses of ACV

This chapter is all about showing you other ways to use apple cider vinegar in your daily life.

Below are a number of ways you can start using ACV right away. They're simple, effective and low cost!

<u>Bug Spray</u>

You can use ACV with essential oil and witch hazel to make an effective bug spray that can be applied directly to the skin. Because this is all natural, you won't be exposing yourself to harmful chemicals like DEET.

There is a quote from the *Scientific American* (<u>https://www.scientificamerican.com/article/is-it-true-that-the-deet/</u>) regarding the mixed research DEET has gotten.

"Duke University pharmacologist Mohamed Abou-Donia, in studies on rats, found that frequent and prolonged DEET exposure led to diffuse brain cell death and behavioral changes, and

concluded that humans should stay away from products containing it. But other studies have shown that while a few people have sensitivity to DEET applications, most are unaffected when they use DEET products on a sporadic basis according to the instructions on the label."

In my opinion, it's better to be safe than sorry. Brain cell death is just not okay in my book. So, why not try a natural alternative that's inexpensive and helps to kill bacteria while nourishing your skin?

Ingredients you'll need:

- ½ cup ACV

- ½ cup witch hazel

- 10 drops eucalyptus essential oil

- 10 drops of either tea tree oil or rosemary essential oil

- 10 drops of lavender essential oil

- 10 drops of either lemon or lemongrass essential oil

- 1 eight-ounce spray bottle, preferably glass

Directions:

Combine all ingredients and pour into the spray bottle.

Apply anyplace on the body you want protection from bugs. Just be sure you don't apply to the eyes and mouth.

Improves Health of the Gut

One of the great things about ACV is its ability to increase the amount of beneficial bacteria your digestive tract needs. These beneficial bacteria help you by increasing your immune system, digesting your food better and improving the nutritional absorption rate of the foods you consume. Just incorporate up to two tablespoons per day in your diet using methods previously discussed.

Kick Cold Symptoms

We've talked extensively about the bacteria fighting properties of ACV, so I'm sure you understand why it can be a big help if you start feeling a cold coming on. The beneficial bacteria will boost your immune system and help get you back on your feet quicker. Just dilute two tablespoons of ACV in a full glass of water and drink, making sure you haven't surpassed the daily recommended allowance. You'll be helping yourself feel better faster.

Varicose Veins

We hear a lot about the value of proper circulation. In fact, many say it's one of the most important and least addressed issues of the day. One of the most common circulations issues faced by many is varicose veins.

Studies (https://www.ncbi.nlm.nih.gov/pmc/articles/PMC4735895/) have shown that ACV combined with witch hazel and applied in a circular motion, can help to improve circulation and alleviate symptoms.

Poison Ivy Rash

If you've ever gotten into poison ivy, you know how itchy and painful it can be. ACV contains potassium, which can help reduce the swelling, itch and pain caused by poison ivy. Apply a teaspoon of ACV directly to the skin a few times each day until the rash is healed.

Flea Killer

We all love our pets, and the last thing we want to do is expose them unnecessarily to chemical laden flea killers. Try this ACV remedy instead. Mix equal parts water and ACV in a spray bottle and apply to their fur once a day. Do this until the fleas are gone.

Seasonal Allergies

No matter where you live, seasonal allergies have become an issue for almost everyone. ACV can be a great help in relieving some of the symptoms. Since ACV contains healthy bacteria, it can increase your immunity and assist your lymphatic system to drain better and remove the symptoms faster and easier. Try diluting two tablespoons of ACV in a tall glass of water and continue use until you feel better. Remember not to exceed the recommended daily allowance for ACV.

Natural Deodorant

One area of the body that has the reputation of being a breeding ground for bacteria is the armpit. And, as we all know, that can lead to body odor.

ACV contains strong antibacterial properties that make it a great natural deodorant. Just use your fingers or a cotton ball and dab the ACV directly onto the skin under the arm. You'll be neutralizing the odor naturally and feel super fresh.

Warts

Almost everyone has experienced a wart at one time in their life. ACV can be extremely effective here. Soak a cotton ball in ACV, tear off a small portion and cover only the wart (not all the skin around it). Then put a band-aid on it and leave it overnight. You'll have to repeat this several times, but eventually it can cause the wart to fall off and out of your life.

Household Cleaner

This is an age-old use of ACV almost everyone has heard about but may have forgotten. The antibacterial properties in the apple cider vinegar make it perfect for cleaning and killing germs and unwanted bacteria. Just mix equal parts of ACV and water in a spray bottle and start cleaning!

Sunburn Relief

Are you a sun lover? Or maybe you've just overdone your time outside and ended up with a sunburn you didn't plan on. ACV is a great way to soothe and speed the healing of that sunburned skin.

Just add the following to a warm bath and soak. You'll be amazed at how quickly your symptoms subside.

- 1 cup ACV

- ¼ cup virgin coconut oil

- 5-10 drops of lavender essential oil

We've just covered a number of additional ways you can use apple cider vinegar to help improve your life starting today. Now it's time to wrap everything up. We'll do that next.

Conclusion

Now you have the most helpful information I could find on apple cider vinegar. As promised, I've kept it simple and direct. Even a beginner can apply these techniques right away to start living a healthier more natural life.

You've learned how raw apple cider vinegar can help you with:

Weight loss

Diabetes

Acne

Skin Conditions

Heartburn

Damaged hair

Plus, I've included several other uses that almost everyone comes across on a daily basis.

Be sure to try as many as possible of the suggestions you find here. ACV is safe and inexpensive to use. That, combined with its many antibacterial and nutritional benefits, will make it a smart addition to dietary and household routines.

Knowing what to do is extremely important. But applying that knowledge is even smarter. So, keep this book handy and start using what you've learned today!

Book Two:

Baking Soda 101 for Beginners

Introduction

If there is any household product that is more useful than duct tape, it would be baking soda.

You can clean with it, unclog drains, put out fires and even kill fleas with it. It makes you smell better and brightens your teeth. It improves your detergent's ability to clean clothes and helps clear gunk out of swollen nasal passages with sinus irrigation.

The ancient Egyptians used natron, a rudimentary form of baking soda. Natron is a natural mineral that contains nahcolite, or what we call baking soda. They didn't know how to refine the substance and instead dug the mineral out of the ground and used it whole. Their main use was as a cleaning agent, not for baking as we do now.

People at that time used yeast for leavening. Yeast occurs naturally in the air, and if you leave a batter or dough exposed to air where bread has been made, it will start to ferment and rise, but that takes time.

This is one of the reasons matzo bread is so important to the celebration of Passover. It represents the Jews having to flee Egypt before their bread had a chance to rise from the naturally occurring airborne yeasts. If they'd only known they could refine natron and make baking soda, culinary history would be dramatically changed!

In 1791, a French chemist named Nicolas Leblanc come up with a process for making sodium bicarbonate, what we commonly all baking soda. Later in 1846, two New York bakers, Austin Church and John Dwight, built the first manufacturing facility in the United States and started producing baking soda from carbon dioxide and sodium carbonate. Today, baking soda is a household name and you'd be hard-pressed to find a household without it.

Baking soda is an amphoteric, which means it can neutralize both acids and bases. Because of those properties and the safe nature of baking soda, many laboratories keep it around in case of a spill. For that same reason, it has come to be a "go to" product for solving everyday household needs, which we'll be discussing later in the book.

Now let's move on to some easy, practical uses for baking soda. Since almost everyone has a sincere desire for a beautiful smile, let's start there.

Chapter One

Baking Soda for Whitening Teeth

In this chapter we're going to discover several ways to safely remove stains from teeth with baking soda.

Today people want to look their best. Most people want to give a good impression to others, as well as feel confident and secure in their appearance. One of the first things people notice about you is your smile. And having beautiful white teeth is a part of a beautiful smile.

The mildly abrasive nature of baking soda is what makes it an effective teeth whitening agent. It works best for surface stains and can prevent discoloration. For deeper stains you may need to see your dentist.

Be sure to use baking soda responsibly or you could end up with dental problems. Continuous overuse could cause damage to the tooth enamel. But, if you use baking soda remedies for teeth whitening responsibly, excellent results can be had. Here are several ways that work well for many people. Choose which works best for you.

Option One: In this option, you'll be using coconut oil with baking soda. Be sure to use virgin coconut oil so you get the good bacteria-fighting lauric acid. Processed coconut oil has had the lauric acid taken out of it, so the bacteria-fighting agent is lost.

When you combine virgin coconut oil and baking soda, you get a safe teeth whitening agent that will also help to improve your oral health.

To do this, combine one tablespoon of baking soda with one tablespoon of virgin coconut oil. Mix this together thoroughly until you get a nice paste, then brush for about two minutes and rinse thoroughly. This option can be used two or three times a week, and in a few months with regular use, you can see a nice difference in the color of your teeth.

Option Two: With this option you'll be mixing baking soda with your regular toothpaste. This is another safe choice. The fluoride present in most toothpastes helps to strength the enamel while fighting cavities, and the mild abrasive action of the baking soda will help get rid of stains and discoloration. You'll get better results if you use a white toothpaste vs. a fancy gel.

To try this, put a little baking soda into a small bowl and add twice as much toothpaste. Mix that together to make a paste, then brush for two minutes and rinse well after. Do this once or twice a week for a few months and notice the changes you get.

Option Three: I found this to be a little surprising, but it actually works. Here you'll be combining baking soda, salt and strawberries. Even though strawberries are a bright red, the ascorbic acid in them acts as a bleaching agent.

When combined with a pinch of salt and baking soda, you get an effective teeth whitening combination.

Take precaution with this method due to its higher acid nature. Limit the use of this option to twice a month to protect tooth enamel and gums.

Here's what to do. Mash two or three large strawberries with a fork, add one tablespoon of baking soda and mix. Sprinkle in a pinch of salt and mix again. Now brush with the resulting paste for about two minutes and rinse thoroughly. Repeat every two weeks for a few months.

Option Four: This method uses hydrogen period mixed in with the baking soda. Hydrogen peroxide is a safe bleaching agent commonly used for teeth whitening and helps kill harmful bacteria. When you combine hydrogen peroxide and baking soda, free radicals will be released that go to work breaking up the stain molecules sitting on the surface of your teeth. Once broken up, those stains are then brushed away.

To do this, mix one tablespoon of baking soda with enough 3% hydrogen peroxide to make a paste in a small bowl. Be sure to mix them together thoroughly until the paste is smooth. Then brush your teeth with the paste for about two minutes and rinse thoroughly. Do this twice a week for eight to ten consecutive weeks to get noticeable results.

If you notice this paste mixture is too strong for your teeth and gums, add equal portions of water and hydrogen peroxide to the baking soda. That will water down the strength of the hydrogen peroxide. If needed, play around with the amounts of water and hydrogen peroxide until you find the right strength for you.

Option Five: This is one of the simplest ways. Simply mix a tablespoon of baking soda with enough water to make a paste and carefully brush your teeth for two minutes. Be sure to rinse thoroughly. Repeat this process once a week for several months to achieve noticeable results.

Option Six: This method uses lemon juice mixed with baking soda. Lemon juice is found in a variety of home remedies and most people have lemons or lemon juice readily available in their homes.

It's the citric acid in lemon juice that makes it a good bleaching agent and can produce good results with just one treatment. But it's also very strong and shouldn't be used more than once every two to three months. If you choose to use this combination more often, dilute the lemon juice down with equal amounts of water. But be responsible and don't overdo it. Such limited use shouldn't produce any dental issues, but you can always check with your dentist first if you have any questions.

This is the procedure. Put a teaspoon of lemon juice and a teaspoon of baking soda in a small bowl and mix it into a paste. You'll notice the fizzing will decrease the more you stir. Now brush for no more than two minutes and be sure you completely rinse out all traces of the mixture. Don't leave any of it behind in your mouth. For many, this option gives instant gratification in removing stains from their teeth.

Things to Remember:

- If you have any questions or concerns about any of these options, consult your dentist first before trying them. This also applies if you have sensitive gums or teeth.

- Be sure to keep up regular brushing and oral care. Don't substitute teeth whitening techniques for regular brushing.

- Make the pastes we talked about here as smooth as possible. If the paste is too gritty it could damage tooth enamel.

- If you're wearing braces or a permanent retainer and they use orthodontic glue, don't brush with baking soda as it will soften the glue.

- Only use these processes as instructed above and certainly no more than two or three times a week, depending on the option you choose. Overuse could lead to tooth enamel erosion or cause teeth to become sensitive.

- Don't brush longer than two minutes at a time with these pastes and brush, don't scrub. Harsh scrubbing can damage gums and tooth enamel.

Responsible use of these procedures can save you a lot of money and trips to the dentist. Experiment and find the option that works best for you.

You just learned six different ways of using baking soda to help whiten your teeth. Next, we'll find out how to use baking soda to help combat heartburn.

Chapter Two

Heartburn and Baking Soda

This chapter is all about the role of baking soda in combating heartburn and why it works.

The use of baking soda for heartburn is an old-time remedy most people have forgotten about. Since heartburn is such a difficult problem for so many to live with, the idea it could be addressed using something as simple as baking soda may seem surprising.

Internally, it works like this. Baking soda contains sodium bicarbonate. On the pH scale, bicarbonate is highly basic/alkaline. That makes it somewhat unconventional to start with. Most foods are slightly acidic or very acidic. Ideally, it would be best to eat foods that are neutral on the pH scale. Eating foods too basic or too acidic isn't wise and should be avoided. However, sodium bicarbonate is a very weak base on the pH scale, making it safe in small doses.

Baking soda for heartburn has a clear logic to it. Heartburn is actually a symptom of GERD (gastroesophageal reflux disease). With GERD, the stomach acid pushes up into the esophagus. A weak base like sodium bicarbonate can neutralize that stomach acid, making the pain go away.

Adding ½ to 1 teaspoon of baking soda to a glass of water will normally be enough to neutralize the stomach acid that causes heartburn. People that suffer from chronic heartburn may need to consume this treatment regularly for heartburn relief and see their health care practitioner.

Baking soda for heartburn relief has the added benefit of being inexpensive. A container of this simple household item can last for months, even if used on a regular basis. Antacids, on the other hand, have to be replaced fairly often. And antacids can have side effects like diarrhea or constipation. Consuming large amounts of antacids that contain calcium carbonate can affect the balance of calcium and acid in the body and damage the kidneys.

Sodium bicarbonate is biologically produced by the pancreas to combat stomach acid. Baking soda has few ingredients other than sodium bicarbonate, which means you're not ingesting a host of other chemicals. Using baking soda for heartburn relief is a simple matter of replicating the internal processes that already exist to combat excess stomach acid in the first place.

Keep in mind that baking soda isn't a permanent solution for chronic heartburn. Consult your medical practitioner if that's what's happening to you.

We just learned how baking soda helps to quickly and inexpensively relieve heartburn. Now let's learn how to safely use and not use baking soda.

Chapter Three

Use Baking Soda Responsibly

In this chapter we'll cover how much baking soda to take and who should not be using it due to medical conditions.

How to Take

Baking soda is easy to use. Adults and teens can dissolve 1/2 teaspoon in four or more ounces of water. Be sure it's completely dissolved before drinking. This dosage can be repeated in two hours if needed.

For children, the dosage should be determined by your doctor.

Normally you wouldn't want to take more than 3.5 teaspoons of baking soda in a day. If you're over 60, you'd wouldn't want to take more than 1.5 teaspoons per day.

If you find you're needing the maximum dosage for at least two weeks, you should see your health care practitioner as you may have a more serious condition. You don't want to exceed the maximum dosage for more than two weeks.

Be sure to take your time when drinking baking soda for stomach upset. If you drink it too fast, it could lead to increased diarrhea and gas. Also, don't take baking soda if you're overly full.

Always remember that too much baking soda can cause an increase in acid production, or acid rebound, and make symptoms worse. Be sure the baking soda is completely dissolved in a minimum of four ounces of water and sip it slowly.

Baking soda has many great advantages and is well tolerated by most people. But, just like anything else, it's not for everyone and needs to be used responsibly. Below are a few things to consider before using baking soda.

The Skin

If you have highly sensitive skin, you're likely to find bathing in baking soda irritating. The skin is the body's largest organ and is slightly acidic. That helps moisture cling to the skin and keep the bad bacteria out. So, if you have sensitive skin, you may find the alkaline nature of baking soda isn't for you when it comes to a soak in the tub.

The Hair

Some people make up a mixture of baking soda and apple cider vinegar and use that as a cleanser for their hair instead of shampooing. Occasional use is fine and won't be a problem; but excessive use over time isn't a good idea. The scalp and hair are naturally acidic. An occasional use of baking soda may make your hair shine, but too much use over time can cause breaks and frizzing.

Athletic Performance

You may have heard about athletes drinking a large amount of baking soda before an event to increase endurance. These types of aids are known as ergogenic. The basic idea is fairly straight forward. Since hard exercise makes your muscles and blood more acidic, baking soda can partially counteract that and theoretically let you exercise harder longer.

Several studies have been done and results are varied. There can be a small boost in performance for short events under ten minutes. But, loading baking soda can also cause gastrointestinal side effects like explosive diarrhea when taken too often and in excess.

Avoid High Doses in General

Like most everything out there, over-consumption is not advised. It can cause irritability, headache and nausea. If any of these conditions persist, consult your medical practitioner. Also, if you develop any other conditions that are unusual for you, let your medical practitioner know what you're experiencing.

Other Precautions

- If you're taking prescription medications, consult a pharmacist or your doctor before use. A few antacid type products may interfere with some medications.
- Do not take baking soda if you are on a sodium restricted diet unless you consult your doctor first.
- Don't give to children under five years of age without careful consideration.
- Make sure baking soda is completely dissolved before taking it.
- Don't take baking soda when you're overly-full from eating and drinking.
- Consult your medical professional if severe stomach pain occurs after consuming baking soda.

Although most of these items are common-sense, it's always good to review and remember them.

While I've covered many of the most common contraindications, there may be others that could apply to your situation. Be sure to consult your medical practitioner with any questions and follow-up with your own research before undertaking any new health care regimen.

We've just discussed how much baking soda to take, how to take it and when not to use baking soda. Next, we're going to discuss how baking soda can help with acne and scars.

Chapter Four

Acne and Scars

In this chapter we talk about two big topics in skin care, acne and scars, and how baking soda can help.

Simple is beautiful. When it comes to acne home applications, and you can't get simpler than baking soda. It's a great natural solution. Plus, it's very inexpensive when compared to other skin care products available on the market.

I'm sure you know that acne forms when bacteria grows in skin pores that are blocked by excess sebum and dead skin cells. The immune system attacks the bacteria, and this causes inflammation and leads to red and painful pimples. Proper use of baking soda can help you keep skin pores open and free from acne causing bacteria.

Bacteria in general, blossom in acidic settings. Baking soda is basic or alkaline. It can kill acne causing bacteria by neutralizing the acidity they require.

Be sure to do a skin test first, especially if you have sensitive skin. To test, apply a paste of baking soda and water on the inside of your wrist and wait a few minutes. If your skin starts to flush or itch, then skip using baking soda for skin care.

If your test goes well, try some of these effective ways to help your skin with blemishes.

Face Masks

A baking soda mask for acne is a simple process but produces excellent results. Combine baking soda and water to make a paste, making sure it isn't too runny. Then apply the paste to your face for fifteen minutes and wash off. This will make the skin look fresh and remove any pore clogging debris. Normally, you'd want to do this before going to bed, four times each week.

Like most home acne solutions, don't forget to wash your face before applying any of these treatments. Avoid rubbing your face with a towel when you dry. Instead, pat your face dry.

Spot Treatment

This method is similar to the first. Once you make the paste of baking soda and water, use a cotton swab and dab it onto the pimple itself. It can be left on overnight by doing it this way and washed off in the morning. Baking soda has the capacity to dry out the blemish and remove the trapped oils. As we discussed earlier, always wash your face before and after and pat dry.

Start Out Slowly

Don't move into these routines too quickly. Even if you're anxious to get rid of your acne, take your time to implement what we've discussed. Baking soda can irritate your skin if it's too sensitive. Start with once or twice a week and see how your skin reacts to these treatments. Later, you can use them more often when you're sure they're a match for your skin type.

If you find you'd like a more potent treatment, try mixing a drop of neem or tea tree oil into your baking soda paste. Both of these oils are anti-bacterial and antiseptic and will help to combat the acne causing bacteria.

Scars

Baking soda has been used for years to help diminish the appearance of scars. It is a natural exfoliant, so it gently scrapes away the scar tissue layer by layer. Remember, this is a slow process, and you won't see a scar diminish overnight.

To use, begin by making a light paste of one-part baking soda and two-parts water. Gently scrub the scar area for a minute. Be sure not to over-scrub during the treatment. Then rise and apply vitamin E oil to keep the area soft and replenish oils that were scrubbed away by the baking soda.

Vitamin E may also help to fade the scar out over time.

We just covered how to help rid yourself of acne and scars using baking soda. Next, we'll go over ways to use it to clean your home.

Chapter Five

A Clean Home

This chapter is all about your home and how you can help keep it clean safely and naturally.

Baking soda is great when it comes to common household cleaning shores. In an era where we're exposed to so many toxic chemicals, it's nice to know something as mild as baking soda can also be effective.

Here are some uses you can start using today.

For Drains

I've long used baking soda and white vinegar for drain maintenance. It's the perfect solution to keeping kitchen and bathroom drains clean and fresh smelling. Just put a teaspoon or less of baking soda into the drain and then pour in about a tablespoon of vinegar. You may want to experiment to find what works best in your sinks.

Smart small though. The combination of baking soda and vinegar causes an active fizzing and bubbling.

It's this bubbling process that tells you if the box of baking soda you've had around forever is still good, too. If your baking soda is still good, it will bubble away merrily!

If your drain is clogged, try using a lot more baking soda. One recipe is to pour a cup of baking soda down the drain, then a cup of vinegar. Wait several minutes, then run hot water and see if you've cleared the drain. If not, repeat the process, but wait longer to flush afterward with the hot water, possibly even overnight.

Remove Odors

A well-known use of baking soda is to keep an open box in the refrigerator to neutralize odors. Because baking soda clears odor, it can also be put in the bottom tray of an oven-type electric toaster to reduce the burnt smells. Some use it to eradicate smells in bottles or jars that milk or other liquids have left an odor in. Be creative... where there's a smell, use baking soda!

Scrubbing Agent

Baking soda is an abrasive that is milder than commercial cleansers, but still very effective. Use it to scrub out the sink, bathtub or shower stall. Just pour baking soda onto a rag or sponge, add a little water on top to form a paste and scrub.

You can also mix up the paste in a small cup or bowl and throw out what you haven't used at the end of the cleaning session or put it to use scrubbing dishes.

Some people like to keep a small container of baking soda in a closed jar by the sink so it's handy. You can also put it in a salt shaker and dispense it that way. You'll probably go through it so quickly you won't have to be concerned about it caking. If you do notice caking in the salt shaker, add a few grains of rice to the baking soda to absorb any moisture and that should alleviate the problem.

Pots and pans that have been burned on the bottom call for sterner measures. Make a baking soda paste with water and apply it generously over the burned area, letting the pot sit overnight. In the morning, reapply a fresh layer of paste and scrub.

Carpet Odors

Over a period of time, carpets can begin to smell. With pets and children in the house, there can be concerns about using carpet cleaners that are chemical laden. Baking soda can do a great job to lift dirt and odor without that worry.

If you have smelly carpets or area rugs caused by pets or even general use, then baking soda should be able to help you out. Baking soda has odor neutralizing qualities and as it penetrates deep into the carpet fibers, it will absorb any odor that might be present.

Sprinkle an even layer of baking soda on your dirty carpet and leave it overnight to neutralize odor. In the morning, vacuum it up. You'll notice how fresh and clean the carpet smells as soon as you finish vacuuming.

<u>For a really deep carpet cleaning, try this:</u>

Use a shaker jar to spread baking soda over your carpet. Be sure to apply corner-to-corner in an even systematic manner. Begin in one corner of the room and liberally sprinkle the baking soda on the carpet. Try to cover a 3x3 foot section at a time and use enough baking soda so you can barely see the color of the carpet through the baking soda.

Then use a toothed brush or broom or even a wide-toothed comb and brush the baking soda into the carpet so it sinks into the fibers.

Continue this process until the entire room is done.

Now let that sit for a few hours. Try to limit any activity in the area, as constantly walking on it will lessen the cleaning effect the baking soda will have.

Next vacuum your carpet thoroughly. Start by working on one small section at a time, vacuuming in one direction, then at a 90-degree angle, to extract the baking soda from deep within the carpet fibers.

This is a rather involved process, but the end result is well worth it, and can save a lot of money.

Carpet Stains

You can also get rid of carpet stains by using baking soda.

Mix ¼ cup of baking soda with two teaspoons of white vinegar to make a paste. Apply it to the soiled area and let it dry overnight. The next day, use a soft bristle brush to remove the hardened paste, then vacuum. You should have removed the stain completely with this process. If it's really stubborn, you may need to repeat the process.

Urine in Carpets

We all love our pets, and no matter how well trained they may be, accidents are going to happen.

If you catch it right away, blot up the urine from the carpet immediately. If it sets, the odor will dry into the carpet fibers.

To address this, mix two cups of white vinegar, two cups of warm water and four tablespoons of baking soda and pour that into a spray bottle. Spritz it directly onto the stained area and let it sit for five to ten minutes, then blot it up.

For heavier stains, you'll want to sprinkle baking soda directly onto the spot. Then make a mixture that's 50/50 water and white vinegar and pour that directly on top of the baking soda. Let it sit for five minutes and blot it up with a towel.

Coffee Makers

A great way to clean your coffee or tea maker is with baking soda. Left unchecked, a dirty coffeemaker will make coffee bitter and can cause mold to grow. Aside from the unwanted taste, this can cause gastrointestinal problems like gas, bloating and diarrhea.

To clean the coffee maker parts, make a paste from 1 cup of baking soda and ½ cup water. You may need to experiment with this mixture to get the right consistency. The point is to make a paste you can use to scrub all the coffeemaker parts with. You can use a sponge or soft-bristled brush to help you scrub off rancid oils and get into crevices.

Once you have cleaned all the parts, rinse them thoroughly in warm water. You can also wash them afterward in soapy water to make sure there is no baking soda residue left and then rinse. Your coffee brewer parts should now be squeaky clean.

You'll also want to get rid of any mold that may be growing down inside your coffeemaker where you can't reach. To do this, you'll want to run a baking soda cycle through the coffee or tea maker. This is done by filling your coffee pot with warm water and adding ¼ cup of baking soda. Be sure to use warm water so the baking soda is thoroughly dissolved. Now allow the coffeemaker to run as if it were brewing a pot of coffee.

Once finished, run at least two pots of plain warm water through the coffeemaker to make sure you've flushed out all baking soda residue. This will insure the insides have been thoroughly rinsed.

This is a great procedure to do every week to insure you're keeping your coffeemaker sparkling clean and protecting your health at the same time.

Clean Your Oven

Sprinkle baking soda over the oven and then spray it with water. For oven walls, make a baking soda paste and apply it generously. Let that sit overnight. The next day, scrub the oven with a fresh baking soda and water paste and scoop out the gunk that comes off. Rinse thoroughly.

Mop Floors

Add ½ cup of baking soda to a bucket of warm water and mop. You might need to get a cloth or sponge and scrub scuff marks with a baking soda/water paste to get rid of them. Be sure to rinse thoroughly after.

Grease & Oil Stains

Pour baking soda directly onto these stains and scrub with a web brush. Continue until the spot is gone, then rinse thoroughly.

Walls & Furniture

Any painted surface can be cleaned with baking soda on a damp cloth or sponge. Scrub lightly, rinse and dry with a clean cloth.

We just covered several ways to safely clean your home using baking soda. Next up is the role baking soda plays in dealing with urinary tract infections.

Chapter Six

Urinary Tract Infections

In this chapter we'll discuss how baking soda can help with UTI's.

Did you know that urinary tract infections (UTIs) are the second most common infection plaguing people today? These infections are responsible for 8.1 million visits to health care professionals every year (https://havefiness.com/everything-need-know-utis/). Women in particular are susceptible and 40-50% of women will deal with at least one of these infections in their lifetime. For many women, it is a reoccurring issue (https://www.ncbi.nlm.nih.gov/pubmed/210954 09).

The conventional wisdom is to use antibiotics to treat this infection. E.coli, the primary bacteria that causes UTIs, is becoming more and more resistant to those antibiotics. Fortunately, there are natural solutions to help with this common infection and baking soda is one of them.

A study was published in 2017 (https://www.ncbi.nlm.nih.gov/pubmed/28975365) on the effects of baking soda when used to combat UTIs. The subjects consisted of 33 women with an acidic urine pH lower than six.

In the study the subjects took oral doses of 4 grams (a little less than a teaspoon) of baking soda dissolved in water twice a day for four weeks. After four weeks, researchers tested the urine pH of the test subjects. They found the urine was alkalinized and there was "a significant level of positive effects on symptoms and symptom scores".

While baking soda is not the only answer, the study does show it to be an effective and inexpensive way to deal with UTIs without all the side effects of many prescription medications.

We've just discussed the role baking soda can have in combating urinary tract infections. Next let's talk about how it can help with gout relief.

Chapter Seven

Gout and Baking Soda

This chapter is all about gout; what it is and how baking soda can help.

Gout has become a concern for many people today. When excess uric acid crystallizes in the joints, it's called gout. Those acid crystals have sharp microscopic points and can cause swollen joints, redness and pain and is often associated with arthritis.

The use of baking soda is now getting great reviews among gout sufferers. To help relieve gout, add ½ teaspoon of baking soda to 8 ounces of water. Do this just before bedtime and again in the morning when you get up. Be sure not to exceed the daily recommended dosage of 3.5 teaspoons per day or 1.5 teaspoons per day if you're over 60. When properly done, this treatment can often relieve gout symptoms.

It is recommended that you consult with your medical practitioner first before using baking soda for gout. Your doctor knows your medical history and is aware of other conditions you may have that could be a consideration.

Now that we've discussed how to use baking soda for gout, let's discuss how it can help with thrush.

Chapter Eight

Baking Soda and Thrush

In this chapter we'll cover what thrush is and how baking soda can be a natural way to deal with it.

What is thrush? It's a medical condition where a yeast known as Candida Albicans overgrows in the mouth and throat. This causes white patches inside the mouth, as well as soreness and pain.

Candida is normally present in everyone. It's only a problem when it overgrows and takes over normally healthy tissues. This is the same yeast overgrowth that causes diaper rash on babies.

So, what causes thrush?

There are a number of causes in adults:

- Smoking is at the top of the list by disturbing the natural balance of oral bacteria.

- Dentures can also cause thrush if not taken care of properly. They must be cleaned daily and removed at night.

- Overuse of antibacterial mouthwash is also a culprit. Too much will affect the good bacteria and encourage Candida to overgrow.

- The prolonged use of antibiotics will also disrupt the oral flora which may lead to thrush.

- Prolonged periods of stress are a problem since they weaken the immune system. This prevents the good bacteria from keeping the Candida in check.

- People with immune disorders such as AIDS and cancer are also more susceptible to thrush, as are diabetics.

Here are two simple methods for using baking soda to combat thrush.

1. Mix baking soda and water to form a paste and apply it to the affected areas in your mouth with a cotton swab. Allow it to

sit for a few minutes, then thoroughly rinse your mouth with warm water. This should be done after every meal until you see your symptoms improve.

2. The other method is to dissolve ½ teaspoon of baking soda in a full glass of water. Use this solution to gargle and swish with. Use the full glass of solution, then rinse thoroughly with plain water. Continue doing this until the thrush is gone. This procedure can also be done after the first one discussed above when dealing with patches in the throat or at the back of the mouth that are difficult to help with a spot treatment.

Again, it's always wise to consult your medical practitioner with any questions before beginning a new health regimen.

We just talked about combating thrush with baking soda. Next, we'll find out how to use baking soda in our daily personal care.

Chapter Nine

Personal Care

In this chapter we're going to cover how we can effectively and economically use baking soda instead of expensive personal hygiene products.

We all care about how we look and present ourselves to the outside world. But so many of the personal care and beauty products on the market today come with a high price tag and can be filled with unnatural chemicals.

Many natural beauty products can be created in the convenience of your own home using a box of baking soda and just a few additional ingredients. Here are several natural ideas for your personal care and beauty regimen that won't break the bank.

Bath Retreat

Who doesn't love a soak in a warm relaxing bath? This baking soda bath oil is the perfect thing to enhance that experience.

To do this, you'll need the following ingredients:

- 4 tablespoons of baking soda
- 16 fluid ounces of milk
- 8 fluid ounces of honey
- 16 tablespoons of sea or cooking salt
- 4 fluid ounces of baby oil

Mix the honey, milk, baking soda and salt into a large bowl and stir well. Pour this mixture into a tub of warm water and add the baby oil, using your hands to stir the mixture into the water to distribute it evenly.

Now step into the bath, sit back and enjoy the soothing water while you soak your troubles away.

Foot Care

Try this special treat for those tired neglected feet.

First dissolve 3 tablespoons of baking soda in a tub or basin of warm water and soak your feet for approximately 5 to 10 minutes. Pat your feet dry and move onto the next step.

Now make a paste of baking soda and water and gently exfoliate your feet. You'll feel better all over and your feet will love you.

Skin Exfoliant

Dead surface cells can leave the skin feeling rough and dry. Making your own exfoliant to remove those dead cells is simple. Make a paste of 3-parts baking soda to 1-part water. Rub the paste onto your face or body in a gentle circular motion, then rinse thoroughly with warm water. Now run your hand across your skin and see how smooth it feels.

Nail Care

Using baking soda to soften cuticles and clean nails is easy. Simply apply baking soda to your cuticle brush. Now scrub for great looking nails.

Dry Shampoo

Running late and don't have time to shampoo? Here's a quick trick to try. Mix 1-part baking soda, 1-part baby powder and 3 drops of your favorite essential oil, like lavender. Apply the mixture to the roots of your hair, including the bangs and comb through. The mixture will absorb excess oil and freshen up your hair, giving you just the clean you need until your next shampoo.

Clean Brushes and Combs

Keeping the items we use on our hair clean is an absolute must to having a truly healthy head of hair. This is easy to do using baking soda.

To remove the buildup of oil and hair product residue, soak combs and brushes in a solution of

1 teaspoon of baking soda in a small tub or basin of hot water. The baking soda will help break up the greasy residue and leave combs and brushes smelling fresh. Then rinse them thoroughly and allow them to dry before your next use.

We just covered some of the simple ways to use baking soda in your personal care routines. Next, we'll cover how to use baking soda to deal with issues outside the home.

Chapter Ten

Outdoor Uses

We've been discussing several therapeutic and personal uses of baking soda. But what about problems you may deal with outside the home? We'll cover that next.

<u>Crabgrass</u>

This seems to be a never-ending issue for many people. Crabgrass gets in the way of having that nice uniform green lawn so many strive for. Baking soda can help with this situation.

When you find a patch of crabgrass, sprinkle a little baking soda on it. This will help to kill the crabgrass without resorting to harmful chemicals that are also more expensive.

Walkway Cleaner

Baking soda is a great way to clean sidewalks, patios and decorative rocks in your yard. Put some of the dry baking soda in a pan. Now wet the areas you want to clean, dip a cleaning brush into the dry baking soda and scrub. You'll notice how easily the dirt comes off, leaving you with the clean surface you desire.

Ants & The Sandbox

Kids love to play outside in the sand. But ants can invade their play space and sometimes even bite. To deal with this, mix a box of baking soda into every 40 pounds of sand. This will deter ants and other unwanted insects, all without causing harm to your child.

Caterpillar Problems

While some caterpillars are relatively harmless, there are those that love to invade your garden and eat your vegetables and greens, depriving you of the delicacies you're trying so hard to grow. Simply sprinkle baking soda around the plants. This will help deter the caterpillars, save your plants, and keep you safe from toxic chemicals.

Weeds & Sidewalk Cracks

No one likes to see weeds growing up between the cracks in the sidewalk. They are unwelcome guests and can be a real nuisance. Try sprinkling baking soda on them and see what happens.

Fleas

Fleas can be a real pain to deal with and eliminate. No one wants them moving out of the yard onto them or their pets. Try sprinkling baking soda over your lawn where you're having the problem. The baking soda will dehydrate the fleas and eventually kill them.

We just covered several uses of baking soda for outside the home. Next, we'll cover a variety of baking soda uses to help with even more issues.

Chapter Eleven

Other Various Uses

In this chapter we'll cover a more common problems and how baking soda can help.

Bee Stings & Insect Bites

These are the worst, right? The itching can almost drive you crazy. Here comes baking soda to the rescue. Make a paste of baking soda and water and dab it directly onto the sting or bite. You'll get immediate relief. Let it dry on the affected skin and repeat if necessary. If dealing with a wasp sting, diluted vinegar works better.

Poison Ivy or Chicken Pox

If you've been caught in poison ivy and have a large affected area, soaking in a warm bath with ½ cup of baking soda dissolved in the water will help stop the itch right away. If it's only a small area, you can use a wet baking soda compress.

Since chicken pox can affect the entire body, you'll want to do the baking soda bath soak. This will not only relieve the itching but help the scabs to fall off by themselves into the water without leaving a scar.

Stuffy Nose

This can work wonders. Mix ¼ teaspoon of baking soda in 1 tablespoon of water, making sure you stir to completely dissolve the baking soda. Now tilt your head back and put a drop or two in each nostril.

Chest Congestion

This is an old-time remedy that still works today. Put a teaspoon of baking soda in your vaporizer and deeply breathe in the steam. This will help to clear the mucous and keep the unit clean at the same time.

Sore Throat

There are two different options to try for this.

1. Melt an aspirin in 2 teaspoons of hot water, then add 1 level teaspoon of baking soda and ½ cup of warm water. Now gargle.
2. Mix equal parts of baking soda, brown sugar and salt in a glass of warm water and gargle.

Your Car

Mix ½ cup of baking soda in ½ gallon of warm water. This solution is great for cleaning tires, windows, floor mats and vinyl seats. Be sure to rinse thoroughly.

Litter Boxes

If you have a cat, baking soda is great for absorbing kitty litter smells. Mix a box of baking soda in with the litter and stir thoroughly. You'll notice a difference right away!

Clothes & Shoes

Just like the refrigerator, you can put an open box of baking soda in your closet to absorb odor from shoes and clothes like coats, etc. For really smelly shoes, sprinkle some baking soda directly into them between wearings. Then when ready to wear, shake the baking soda out and wipe with a damp cloth.

We've just gone over several various uses for baking soda. Now let's wrap it all up.

CONCLUSION

I hope you've enjoyed this book on baking soda. I know I've enjoyed writing it for you and sharing the tips and secrets I've picked up over the years.

We've covered a lot of ground and there are so many ways to help yourself and your loved ones with baking soda. It's safe, natural and using it will save a lot of money compared to so many of the products out on the market today.

Are you also interested in coconut oil and what it can do for you while saving money?

Want to make sure you're buying the right kind of coconut oil? And how it can triple your metabolism to help burn off the fat while boosting your brain at the same time? Then visit my website: CoconutOilBreakthrough.com.

If you'd like to stay in touch with me, you can reach me on my Facebook page at

https://www.facebook.com/BJ.Richards.Author/
or at my website, bjrichardsauthor.com.

Have a happy, healthy life!

Made in the USA
Middletown, DE
14 April 2020

89311665R00071